2,1.94

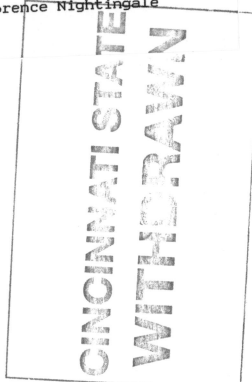

FLORENCE NIGHTINGALE

Notes on Nursing Theories

SERIES EDITORS

Chris Metzger McQuiston
Doctoral Candidate, Wayne State University

Adele A. Webb
College of Nursing, University of Akron

Notes on Nursing Theories is a series of monographs designed to provide the reader with a concise description of conceptual frameworks and theories in nursing. Each monograph includes a biographical sketch of the theorist, origin of the theory, assumptions, concepts, propositions, examples for application to practice and research, a glossary of terms, and a bibliography of classic works, critiques, and research.

1   **Martha Rogers: The Science of Unitary Human Beings**
    Louette R. Johnson Lutjens

2   **Imogene King: A Conceptual Framework for Nursing**
    Christina L. Sieloff Evans

3   **Callista Roy: An Adaptation Model**
    Louette R. Johnson Lutjens

4   **Dorothea Orem: Self-Care Deficit Theory**
    Donna L. Hartweg

5   **Rosemarie Parse: Theory of Human Becoming**
    Sheila Bunting

6   **Margaret Newman: Health as Expanding Consciousness**
    Joanne Marchione

7   **Paterson and Zderad: Humanistic Nursing Theory**
    Nancy O'Connor

8   **Madeleine Leininger: Cultural Care Diversity and Universality Theory**
    Cheryl L. Reynolds and Madeleine M. Leininger

9   **Florence Nightingale: An Environmental Adaptation Theory**
    Louise C. Selanders

10 **Hildegard E. Peplau: Interpersonal Nursing Theory**
    Cheryl Forchuk

11 **Betty Neuman: The Neuman Systems Model**
    Karen S. Reed

12 **Ida Jean Orlando: A Nursing Process Theory**
    Norma Jean Schmieding

FLORENCE NIGHTINGALE

An Environmental Adaptation Theory

Louise C. Selanders

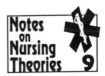

Notes on Nursing Theories 9

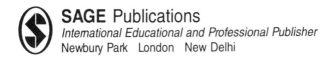

SAGE Publications
International Educational and Professional Publisher
Newbury Park   London   New Delhi

For information address:

SAGE Publications, Inc.
2455 Teller Road
Newbury Park, California 91320

SAGE Publications Ltd.
6 Bonhill Street
London EC2A 4PU
United Kingdom

SAGE Publications India Pvt. Ltd.
M-32 Market
Greater Kailash I
New Delhi 110 048 India

Printed in the United States of America

Library of Congress Cataloging-in-Publication Data

Selanders, Louise C.
    Florence Nightingale: an environmental adaptation theory /
Louise C. Selanders.
        p.   cm. — (Notes on nursing theories; 9)
    Includes bibliographical references.
    ISBN 0-8039-4859-X (cl). — ISBN 0-8039-4860-3 (pb)
    1. Nursing—Philosophy.   2. Nightingale, Florence, 1820-1910.
I. Title.   II. Series: Notes on nursing theories; v. 9.
    [DNLM: 1. Nightingale, Florence, 1820-1910.   2. Nursing Theory.
3. Nurses—biography.   WY 86 S464f   1993]
RT84.5.S45   1993
610.73'01—dc20
[B]
DNLM/DLC   93-28309

93 94 95 96 10 9 8 7 6 5 4 3 2 1

Sage Production Editor: Diane S. Foster

Contents

Foreword, *Raymond G. Hebert*   vii

Preface   ix

Biographical Sketch of the Nurse Theorist   1

1. The Life and Times of Florence Nightingale   3
   The Philosophical Development of Nightingale   3
   Spirituality and Florence Nightingale   8
   The Cultural Context of the Nightingalean Era   9
   Origins of the Model   10
   The Nightingale Fund   10
   Philosophical Assumptions   11

2. Nightingale's Theory of Nursing   14
   Introduction   14
   Person   15
   Environment   17
   Health   19
   Nursing   21
   Nightingale's Model of Nursing   22
   Evaluation of Nightingale's Model of Nursing   23

3. Nightingale Then and Now   25
   Clinical Examples   25
   Nightingale Today   26
   Nightingale and Standards of Nursing Practice   27
   The Legacy of Florence Nightingale   31

References   33

Bibliography   35

About the Author   38

To Florence Nightingale
who has driven, delighted, mystified
and, at times, consumed me

and to Bill, Kate and Aimee with love

Foreword

Florence Nightingale's name and reputation clearly symbolize the nursing profession. Few would doubt the claim that any other name is as well known as hers to modern nurses. Yet, if asked, few would be able to offer much information about Nightingale's life, particularly beyond the Crimean War. Even fewer could add anything at all about Nightingale and nursing theory.

This book by Dr. Louise C. Selanders is determined to correct this deficiency by combining a succinct but well-crafted summary of Florence Nightingale's life and legacy with an interpretive and useful analysis of her nursing theory and its meaning. The comparison to the American Nurses' Association most recent *Standards of Nursing Practice* is particularly relevant. This analysis effectively demonstrates that Nightingale's theory serves uniquely and brilliantly as a model for current practice.

Dr. Selanders also reminds the reader appropriately, that Florence Nightingale's greatest contributions stem not from the Crimean War experience, but from her postwar activities, her prodigious writings, and especially from her determination to create nursing as a profession. In the concluding section, "The Legacy of Florence Nightingale," the author effectively reminds us of the enormous debt the current nursing profession owes to Florence Nightingale—a fact that is often forgotten.

This monograph, then, is a tribute to Florence Nightingale. It is also a tribute to Louise Selanders. As the careful reader will note, Dr. Selanders has only recently completed her dissertation for Western Michigan University: "An Analysis of the Utilization of Power by Florence Nightingale 1856-1872." During the years of research and writing, the author steeped herself in the life, spiritual nature, dreams, and legacy of the remarkable Florence Nightingale. In Dr. Selanders' words, this book is dedicated, "to Florence Nightingale, who has driven, delighted, mystified, and, at times, consumed me."

For those of us who have studied Nightingale in depth, and for the general reader alike, I am sure that this book will be a true testament to what can be learned from a total commitment to a study of an individual such as Nightingale. We thank Dr. Selanders for sharing the fruits of her labors. In short, both the subject and the author remind us, appropriately, to never forget:

Learning the lessons which [Florence Nightingale] offered provides nursing with a wealth of possibility—and a lasting legacy.

RAYMOND G. HEBERT

Preface

The study of Florence Nightingale represents the study of a unique woman in a unique position of power and prestige. One of her many accomplishments included the development of the philosophical base of modern Western secular nursing. The purpose of this volume is to provide the reader with an overview of Nightingale's perceptions of nursing and to demonstrate how this view remains applicable in today's high-tech world.

Florence Nightingale was a prolific writer. At least 12,000 letters, monographs, and books remain available to those wishing to research her life and thoughts in depth. Numerous biographies, drawn from these primary sources, also exist. Therefore Nightingale should not remain a mystery to those practicing nursing; neither should she be shrouded in myth and fiction. Rather, Nightingale should emerge as a complete human being with strengths and weaknesses, likes and dislikes, accomplishments and failures.

In order to assist the reader in sorting out the myth and the reality surrounding Nightingale, an initial chapter has been included that describes her life and times. However, space dictates that this be only a brief overview. Consequently, the reader is encouraged to read Nightingale from the primary sources. Of greatest interest to nurses may be *Notes on Nursing: What It Is and Is Not* (1859/1946) and

Sick Nursing and Health Nursing (1893/1949), which together describe the nucleus of her thoughts regarding the profession.

The reader is encouraged to apply cultural context when reading the concepts and assumptions of Nightingale. Nineteenth century England represented a world that was vastly different from today's society in the United States. Gender and class dictated the expectations for and goals of the population. Much less was known of the world in which they lived.

Finally, the reader is encouraged to remember that the development of the philosophical base of nursing and nursing education represents only a portion of the accomplishments that Nightingale achieved in her lifetime. Nursing came under the larger umbrella of improving public well-being and standards of hygiene and sanitation. If more people felt and worked as passionately as Nightingale did about improving their world, what a magnificent showcase of accomplishment it would be.

I would like to acknowledge and thank Ray Hebert for his comments and discussion. His insight has continued to make this project worthwhile. I would also like to thank the students of the Michigan State University College of Nursing who have provided a continual source of stimulation and encouragement. It is my intent that this volume provide them with a valuable resource and the stimulus to study modern nursing from its origin.

—LOUISE C. SELANDERS

Biographical Sketch of the Nurse Theorist:
Florence Nightingale

Born: May 12, 1820 in Florence, Italy

Education: Privately educated in the classical mode with
emphasis on languages, literature, philosophy, history,
and mathematics.

Nursing education briefly obtained at Kaiserswerth in
Germany during 1850 and 1851.

Achievements: Superintendency of the London Institution for
the Care of Sick Gentlewomen in Distressed
Circumstances; Superintendent of English nurses in the
Crimean conflict; reform of English Army Medical
School; establishment of military statistics; establishment
of formalized nursing education at St. Thomas' Hospital,
London; reform of hygienic standards for India;
publication of more than 200 books and monographs.

Awards: Order of Merit

Died: August 13, 1910 in London. Consistent with
Nightingale's wishes, she was buried in the family plot in
East Wellow. There are no direct descendents of the
Nightingale family.

1

The Life and Times of Florence Nightingale

The Philosophical Development of Nightingale

During a life that spanned slightly more than 90 years, Florence Nightingale gained recognition for her accomplishments in sanitary and social reform. Her most recognized achievement was the establishment of the principles for modern nursing education and practice. Nightingale's life demonstrated continuing development of the principles that directed her toward goal achievement.

Early Life and Education

The life of Florence Nightingale was one of privilege associated with family wealth set in pre- and Victorian England. Born May 12, 1820 in Florence, Italy, she was named for the city of her birth.

Miss Nightingale was the second daughter and last child of William Edward and Frances Smith Nightingale. Both parents were of wealthy backgrounds that allowed them to provide an upper-class standard of living for their children. This included frequent travel, a classical education, and social prominence. As a result, Miss Nightingale became well traveled and known for her linguistic and mathematical skills. In addition, she was conversant in history, economics, and the arts (Palmer, 1977).

The original family name was Shore. Upon the impending inheritance of the family estate of Lea Hurst in Derbyshire from his mother's uncle, William assumed the name of Nightingale in order to fulfill the terms of the will (Keen, 1982). Lea Hurst was considered too small by Victorian standards (15 bedrooms); it was cold and difficult for entertaining. Consequently, the second family estate of Embley Park in Hampshire in southern England was purchased.

Befitting the English gentry lifestyle, the Nightingale family lived a life of convenience. Time spent at the two estates, combined with extensive annual stays in London, provided the environment of Nightingale's childhood. The family entertained frequently, was considered socially prominent, and introduced Florence and her sister, Parthenope, to politicians, social reformers, and intellectuals of the period. At age 19, Florence and her sister were presented at court (Woodham-Smith, 1953).

Nightingale's parents were diverse in their beliefs and values. Her father was university educated and a supporter of Parliamentary reform (Allen, 1981). He valued education and saw to it that his daughters were tutored in the classics, an advantage not offered many women.

Encouraged by her father, Florence became a capable student, excelling in her studies and demonstrating a real thirst for knowledge. She maintained a close relationship with her father that continued until his death in 1874 (Cook, 1913).

Nightingale's mother was the antithesis of her father. Considered to be very beautiful and an expert at entertaining, Fanny was primarily interested in maintaining social stature and seeing that her daughters married well. Throughout her life, Fanny maintained a close relationship with Parthenope, who seemed to share her mother's goals and ambitions.

Fanny was never supportive of Florence's nursing efforts. Nursing was not considered a suitable occupation for a young lady of stature. Nightingale's mother did not seem to understand her younger daughter's need for independence, either as a child or later as an adult.

In Florence, one is able to see a mixture of the characteristics of her parents. Her father taught her to be scholarly and to use educated arguments; from her mother she learned drive and ambition.

Despite the privilege and travel of Nightingale's early life, these years were marked by periods of depression, illness, family discord, and disenchantment with her lifestyle. Nightingale perceived a need to be productive and useful and did not find entertaining or the rigors of society to be fulfilling. At an early age, she began to care for the family pets. Soon she was called to care for servants on the family estates who were ill or had been injured.

As early as 1844, at the age of 24, Miss Nightingale determined that her profession should be nursing (Cook, 1913). This decision brought family turmoil, not only because Florence wanted to work, but also because of the prevailing reputation of secular nurses. They were felt to be uneducated women of questionable character who sought refuge caring for patients in private homes and hospitals in order to receive room and board. Nurses were stereotyped in the literature by characters such as the drunken Betsy Prig and Sairy Gamp in Charles Dickens's (1986) *Martin Chuzzlewit*.

Miss Nightingale attempted, on several occasions, to receive formalized training in nursing. In 1850, and again in 1851, she was able to spend brief periods at Kaiserswerth on the Rhine in Germany, a Protestant institution that trained Deaconesses in child care and nursing. These two periods represent the only formalized nursing training received by Nightingale (Cook, 1913; Woodham-Smith, 1953).

Nursing in London

In 1853, Miss Nightingale negotiated and obtained the position of Superintendent of Nurses at the Institution for the Care of Sick Gentlewomen in Distressed Circumstances located in London (Vicinus & Nergaard, 1990; Woodham-Smith, 1953). Although she received no pay for this position and became responsible for her own expenses, this employment situation represented the first time she was able to display her skills in nursing and nursing administration.

Miss Nightingale brought about an upgrade in the standards of the nurses and nursing care, expecting that care be based on compassion, observation, and knowledge (Woodham-Smith, 1953). She also designed changes in the building that improved efficiency. These changes included a dumbwaiter to carry trays to and from the basement, hot and cold running water on all floors, and a system of patient call lights. Feeling that her job was complete after a year, she was seeking employment elsewhere when she was called into government service during the Crimean War (Woodham-Smith, 1953).

The Crimean War

By any standard, the Crimean War was neither a well-planned nor a productive conflict. It was fought primarily between Russia and Turkey to gain control over the port of Constantinople, the Eastern Mediterranean, and the overland route to the Eastern trading areas. Great Britain entered the war with France on the side of Turkey in 1854 (Seaman, 1956).

The British were based at Scutari in Turkey, although the fighting occurred in Southern Russia on the Crimean Peninsula. As a result of this location, the wounded and sick had to be transported by ship across the Black Sea nearly 300 miles (Goldie, 1987). The mortality rate approached 60% for the sick and wounded who survived the trip to the Barrack Hospital (Baly, 1988). The British public was alerted to these conditions by the news reporting of correspondent William Howard Russell for the *London Times* (Goldie, 1987).

A public outcry over the plight of the British soldier caused the British government to seek resolution of this problem. It was during this time that the Secretary for War, Sir Sidney Herbert, contacted Miss Nightingale and requested that she and a group of women travel to the Crimea to provide nursing services (Adams & Foster, 1981). Nightingale departed for Turkey with 38 women on October 21, 1854, disembarking at Scutari on November 4 (Cook, 1913).

During the next 21 months, despite resistance from the medical establishment, Nightingale worked to establish hygienic standards in the care of the wounded (Cope, 1958). She insisted that soldiers be bathed, their wounds dressed, and unspoiled food be fed to the sick. A pure water supply was established. As a result of Nightingale's efforts, the mortality rate declined to approximately 2% (Kalisch & Kalisch, 1986).

It should be noted that throughout Nightingale's life she remained absolutely opposed to the notion of germ theory, even though recent discoveries had provided evidence to the contrary (Baly, 1988; Vicinus & Nergaard, 1990). Although many of her reforms proved effective because of the reduction of contagion, she maintained that it was the general introduction of hygienic standards that brought about the improved conditions.

Nightingale returned to England in 1856 at the conclusion of the war. She was sick and exhausted after nearly dying from a bout of Crimean Fever—probably typhus (Veith, 1990). Much to her amazement and dismay, she was a heroine, a status she both disliked and shunned.

The Productive Years

Following her return from the Crimea, Miss Nightingale began her most productive period relative to establishing reform and creating change (Selanders, 1992). By 1872 she had reformed the Army Medical School, established the importance of accurate record-keeping and the need for governmental statistics, developed new systems of purveyance for wartime conditions, and helped to establish standards of hygiene and public health in India. However, her most enduring change was the establishment of formalized secular nursing education.

Miss Nightingale selected St. Thomas' Hospital in London as the site for the Nightingale School. This effort was supported by the Nightingale Fund, monies given by the grateful British public for the service Nightingale had rendered in the Crimea. The school opened in 1860 with approximately 10 students (Baly, 1988).

As a result of Nightingale's influence, she was able to define the nature of nursing clearly and how nursing was distinctly different from, but not subservient to, medicine. This effort began the establishment of nursing as a profession with a sound and specific educational base (Nightingale, 1859/1946; 1893/1949).

Nightingale wrote prolifically. *Notes on Nursing: What It Is and Is Not*, her best known work, was first published in 1859. Designed as a general reference for all persons who might care for another and not as a nursing text, it remains perhaps the most widely known and read volume of nursing literature.

The Later Years

Following the creation of her major reforms and the establishment of The Nightingale School at St. Thomas', Nightingale's health declined and she rarely left her apartment on South Street in London (Veith, 1990). However, she did continue to write, receive visitors, and offer advice in those areas in which she was considered an expert.

It has been hypothesized that her invalid state allowed her to continue to be productive without social pressures (Pickering, 1974). Individuals sought Nightingale's advice without demanding her appearance at social functions.

In 1893 a speech, which clearly defined Nightingale's beliefs regarding the nature of nursing, was delivered for her at the Chicago Exposition (Nightingale, 1893/1949). Her influence on nursing education continued as schools modeled after her philosophy began in the United States, Canada, Europe, and in most of Britain's Imperial possessions, including Australia.

In 1907, in recognition of her contributions to the British nation, the first Order of Merit given to a woman was bestowed upon Florence Nightingale. Three years later, at the age of 90, she died in her sleep at her apartment on South Street in London.

Spirituality and
Florence Nightingale

Devotion to God became prevalent in Nightingale's writings at an early age (Calabria, 1990; Cook, 1913; Widerquist, 1992). Throughout her life, Nightingale recorded a series of four experiences in which God called her into His service. The first occurred just prior to her 17th birthday. These experiences seemed to give purpose and direction to her life.

Nightingale's family had roots in both the Church of England (similar to the Episcopal Church in the United States) and in the Unitarian Church. However, Nightingale became critical of established religion stating, "the most frightful crimes which the world has ever seen have been perpetuated 'to please God' " (Calabria, 1990, p. 68). Consequently she rarely practiced organized religion in her adult years, preferring to believe in a Supreme Being who was perfect and eternal (Widerquist, 1992). In addition, she believed that God developed laws that governed the order of the universe. She later applied these laws to nursing, stating that nursing must place the patient in the best possible condition for Nature [God] to act (Nightingale, 1859/1946).

Certain elements of Nightingale's religious beliefs can be seen in her philosophical development. Central to her value system were her work ethic and the potential for the perfection of humankind. These philosophical beliefs played heavily in the development of a basis for nursing practice.

While Nightingale was superintendent of the Institution for Gentlewomen in London, a requirement existed that patients must be members of the Church of England in order to receive care. Nightingale rapidly removed this requirement, stating that religious affiliation should not be a requirement for receiving health care.

A similar situation existed when Nightingale began to determine the requirements for those who would enter nursing education. At the time that the Nightingale School was being developed, nursing education of a sort did exist. Virtually all schools of nursing were in religious institutions, such as Kaiserswerth, and religious affiliation was required for admission.

Nightingale believed that education should be open to women of all beliefs, just as all patients should be cared for regardless of their religious beliefs. Consequently, there was no religious affiliation requirement for admission to the Nightingale School. While Nightingale is credited as being the founder of modern Western nursing education, more correctly, she should be credited as the founder of modern Western secular nursing.

The Cultural Context of the Nightingalean Era

In order to appreciate the accomplishments of Florence Nightingale fully, it is necessary also to understand the age in which she lived and the cultural expectations of the period. During the Victorian era, England had a classed culture with great differences in the expectations of the education, productivity, and social behavior between the rich and the poor. This period followed the Industrial Revolution. Consequently, the cities had seen great population influxes and the proliferation of manufacturing.

Many new scientific discoveries, including Jenner's smallpox immunization and Priestley's isolation of oxygen, established the basis for medical innovation (Williams, 1987). Church reform gave greater religious freedom of choice (Schultz, 1992). In general, the time offered a more open society than had previous centuries.

Although reform marked the character of the 19th century, it should be remembered that British society was clearly restricted by gender. Women of social prominence were not expected to contribute in any significant fashion to society. Although many could read, educational opportunities were severely restricted for women when compared to their male counterparts. Nightingale's reforms are all the more impressive because of the conditions under which they occurred. Only a woman of single-minded purpose and resolve could have brought about such change.

Origins of the Model

On Nightingale's return from the Crimea in 1856, she perceived a great need for change. During the next 15 years she brought major reform to the British Army and its medical education system as well as establishing the philosophical base for modern nursing education and practice. The changes brought to nursing constitute her most enduring reform.

The watershed event that greatly influenced Nightingale's perception of nursing was her experience in the Crimea. Although she had been aware of the need for hygienic care in England, the Crimea served to magnify the need for sanitary reform.

An integral component of creating this change was the development of a formalized standard for the education of nurses. Although nursing education was not her first priority upon returning from the Crimea, it became something that literally occupied the remainder of her life.

The Nightingale Fund

The Nightingale Fund consisted of monies donated by a grateful British public to be put at Nightingale's disposal and used in whatever manner she saw fit. The entirety of this fund was used to establish the Nightingale School at St. Thomas' Hospital in London.

The Nightingale Fund established the school of nursing as financially independent from the hospital. This financial independence allowed Nightingale, with the authority of the school's governing body, to establish curricula and hire a matron. The matron was responsible for the day-to-day running of the school without major influence being exerted by the medical community.

The Fund also provided publicity for nursing. This publicity helped to begin the process in which nursing was established as a legitimate educational opportunity for women. As a result, the image of nursing was improved and the profession eventually opened to all classes of women (Baly, 1988).

Philosophical Assumptions

Assumptions are ideas that are implicit and assumed to be true without empirical testing (Walker & Avant, 1988). The following assumptions provide insight into Nightingale's values and beliefs. Understanding the assumptions helps to provide a focus for studying the nursing model.

Nightingale did not specifically identify the ideas that formed the basis of her understanding of nursing. Rather, the assumptions were drawn from her books and monographs. Nightingale's belief in God, a strong work ethic, and the functional ability and value of women underlie these assumptions.

Nursing Is a Calling

The context of "calling" in this instance had religious overtones. Nightingale's deeply religious beliefs in the existence of "natural laws" reinforced her perceived nature of nursing. She felt that these laws could be discovered and used to help people improve their health and existence.

To Nightingale, a "calling" was consuming in terms of time and commitment. Therefore nursing was more than an occupation, something that one could not put aside even for short periods of time.

Nightingale also believed that the work of nursing was so important that it should be thought of as though it were a religious vow. Nightingale herself declined marriage on several occasions, stating that she could not carry out the rigorous demands of her chosen work and meet the requirements of family life.

Nursing Is an Art and a Science

Nightingale described the profession as an art and a science in her remarks at the Chicago Exposition (1893/1949). Nightingale's concept of nursing as a science was reflected in her mandate that nurses be formally educated. Her own practice demonstrated a grasp of statistics, logic, and laws of health and health practices.

The art of nursing, however, gave the profession both freedom and depth. This aspect allowed and mandated that the nurse act in a creative and proactive fashion. The art of nursing also permitted the nurse to function as an advocate for the patient.

Mankind Can Achieve Perfection

Nightingale believed that people could control the outcomes of their lives. Therefore they could pursue perfection. As related to health care, this meant that people could pursue perfect health. The role of the nurse was to try to provide the environment in which this perfect health could be achieved.

The manner in which perfection could be achieved was through the understanding of Nature's laws. Nightingale believed that each generation moved toward a logical understanding of these universal laws. Ultimately these laws would be understood and readily used by people to benefit their existence.

Nursing Requires a Specific Educational Base

The idea that nurses required specific education was revolutionary in 19th century England. Nightingale's focus on providing nursing education underscored her belief in the value of educating women in general.

Nightingale emphasized the need to blend a mixture of theoretical and clinical experiences as part of the educational package, stating, "Neither can it [nursing] be taught by lectures or by books [alone] although these are valuable accessories, if used as such: otherwise what is in the book stays in the book" (Nightingale, 1893/1949, p. 24).

Nursing Is Distinct and Separate From Medicine

Although the physician and the nurse may deal with the same client population, nursing is not to be viewed as subservient to medicine; rather, nursing is aimed at discovering the natural laws that will assist in putting the patient in the best possible condition so that nature can effect a cure.

Nightingale frequently said that nursing was particularly well suited for women. This idea appears to be tied to the gender expectations of the 19th century. Given Nightingale's progressive nature, it is unlikely she would uphold this restriction in today's social environment.

Nightingale's ability, determination, and articulation of the philosophical basis of nursing have endured. Most of her broad beliefs and values continue to hold true in nursing practice a century after they were written.

2

Nightingale's Theory of Nursing

Introduction

Each discipline identifies certain phenomena that help to define the nature of the discipline. These concepts remain constant even though a number of different conceptual models or theories may be built around the designated phenomena. These concepts are known as the metaparadigm of a discipline.

The metaparadigm provides a general and consistent perspective for a discipline to develop and to make comparisons among its several conceptual models (Fawcett, 1984). In nursing, the common phenomena around which the discipline has been built are person, environment, health, and nursing (Fawcett, 1984; Fitzpatrick & Whall, 1983; Torres, 1990).

Nightingale did not specifically write in terms of a metaparadigm, nursing theory, or a conceptual model. However, she has been credited with developing the first conceptual model of nursing. Nightingale was a prolific writer. Today, more than 150 monographs and books, as well as over 12,000 letters, provide us with a rich legacy of her thoughts and ideas. All of the necessary elements for the description of a nursing theory are present in these documents.

Person

Person is the recipient of nursing care. In the case of Nightingale, person was generally viewed as being an individual, although families occasionally were the focus of nursing care. Individuals were usually called "patients" in Nightingale's writings.

On multiple occasions Nightingale made it clear in her writings that nurses were to care for patients, not diseases. She agreed with a physician who stated, "I do not treat pneumonia, I treat the person who has pneumonia" (Nightingale, 1893/1949, p. 24).

People were viewed as multidimensional; that is, they were composed of biological, psychological, social, and spiritual elements. The interrelationship of these components encompassed holism.

The biological component of people was addressed in relation to the cure and prevention of disease. People were seen as having reparative powers and nursing should assist these powers as the means of returning people to health. However, illness also could be prevented through the provision of the proper environment in which people should live.

The psychological component was composed of things that defined thought processes, self-concept, feelings, and intellect. In *Notes on Nursing* (1893/1946), Nightingale warned about the lack of variety and the degree of monotony found in most patient's environments. In addition, she stated that the lack of variety could impede healing and may actually cause psychological disease processes.

The social element of people consisted of interactions within society. Nightingale appears to have addressed this concept less directly than the other elements; however, she was aware that patients should not be isolated from others. Nightingale did advise against the practices of idle chatter and offering advice to patients.

The spiritual element of people referred to the value systems that assisted them in making decisions determining right from wrong. Religion, while an important component to many people, was not to be interpreted as the equivalent of spirituality.

Spirituality is a difficult element to assess as it relates to Nightingale's beliefs. Nightingale's spirituality was intricately tied to her religious belief system, but not to a specific religion. She also felt strongly about the inherent value of people and appeared to assume that the spiritual nature of patients was an assumed element rather than a prerequisite for care.

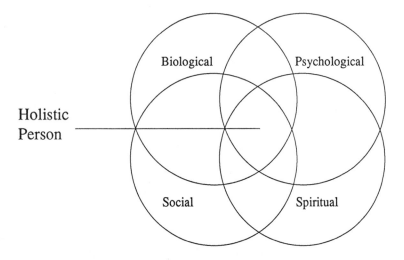

Figure 2.1. Multidimensional Holistic Person

Tied directly to the concept of spirituality was the belief that people were in control of their own destiny. This control was created by making choices in life. The ultimate goal was to move toward perfection (Widerquist, 1992).

The dichotomy of this belief system was that Nightingale was also heavily influenced by the cultural standards of 19th century England, which established rigid rules of social behaviors. Therefore despite the perceived ability of being able to make choices in life, people were expected to obey the cultural norms established by society.

The interaction of these biological, psychological, social, and spiritual elements defines Nightingale's concept of holism. The classical definition of holism states that interacting wholes are more than the sum of their parts (Torres, 1990). Holism implies that an insult to any one of the components effects the entire person to some degree. Therefore people cannot experience a physiological illness such as heart disease without it also affecting their psychological, social, and spiritual components.

This perspective of holism is seen in Figure 2.1. All of the elements appear to have equal value.

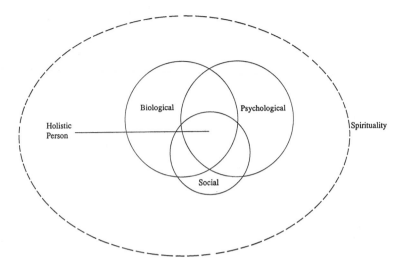

Figure 2.2. Nightingale's Conception of Holism

Nightingale's view of holism appears to be less symmetrical than the classical model. Clearly she did appear to pay more attention to the physical and psychological components than to the other elements of holistic beings. She particularly offers advice in *Notes on Nursing* about various types of physiological care including diet, activity, warmth, light, and care of excrements. Psychological care was also stressed by assuring that patients had variety, an appropriate balance of stimuli and quiet, and that the nurse's behavior did not in any way detract from the patient's environment.

Figure 2.2 more accurately depicts the representation of an holistic individual from Nightingale's perspective. Physiological and psychological needs are seen as predominant, with social needs apparently having less impact on well-being. Spirituality is assumed and pervasive.

Environment

Environment is the core concept in Nightingale's model of nursing. It was her contention that the environment could be altered in such

TABLE 2.1 Nightingale's Major Environmental Elements

Element
Ventilation
Light
Clean Water
Warmth
Noise Control
Management of Wastes and Odors

a way as to improve conditions so that nature could act to cure the patient. The environment consisted of those physical attributes that could be altered and thus improve the patient's well-being.

Nightingale specifically defined elements of the environment that she felt should be monitored and improved when necessary. These are included in Table 2.1.

The most important environmental concerns were ventilation and clean air, followed by clean water. Additional needs that Nightingale identified as critical were provision for warmth, control of noise, provision for light, and adequate management of wastes and odors.

These needs represented chronic problems in Victorian England. The air, especially in the cities, was choked by smoke from burning coal, the chief source of heat. Sanitation was not always well understood. Therefore water supplies were frequently contaminated by human and animal wastes.

Nightingale highlighted these needs as important from a common-sense approach to sanitation. If a clean environment was available to patients, experience told Nightingale that the ability of a patient to survive and eventually recover from disease improved.

In the 1940s, Maslow developed his needs theory. In this theory he identified human needs necessary for human survival. Needs were ordered according to survival priority. Maslow further postulated that lower-level needs had to be met before being able to move to a higher level of need attainment.

Maslow's first-level needs are physiological and included food, air, water, temperature, elimination, and rest. Second-level needs address safety and security issues. Third-level needs are those of social affiliation (Kozier, Erb, & Olivieri, 1991).

A direct comparison can be drawn between Nightingale's perception of human needs within the environment and Maslow's human needs theory. Both address the primary physiological needs, followed by psychological and social needs. Nightingale's perceptions were drawn from empirical observation, and Maslow's theory adds substantiation to her conceptualization.

Nightingale also saw the environment as having external and internal components. She appeared to be as concerned about elements that entered the body—food, water, and medications—as those that directly affected the external body—temperature, bedding, and ventilation (Nightingale, 1859/1946).

Notes on Nursing (1859/1946), Nightingale's most famous publication, was written for the express purpose of informing the general public about how to maintain hygienic conditions within the home and in an illness situation, not as a textbook for nurses. In the preface to *Notes on Nursing*, Nightingale (1859/1946) writes:

> The following notes are by no means intended as a rule of thought by which nurses can teach themselves to nurse, still less as a manual to teach nurses to nurse. They are meant simply to give hints of thought to women who have personal charge of the health of others. Every woman, or at least almost every woman, in England has, at one time or another of her life, charge of the personal health of somebody, whether child or invalid—in other words, every woman is a nurse. (p. 1)

Nightingale did not mean to imply by stating that "every woman was a nurse" that nurses did not require specialized education. Rather, she was stating that nursing is a nurturing art that requires knowledge of sanitary procedures—in essence, how to alter the environment safely. These thoughts were outlined in her 13 canons found in *Notes on Nursing*.

Health

Nightingale (1859/1949) stated that health is "not only to be well, but to be able to use well every power we have to use" (p. 26). Her definition is similar to the World Health Organization's (1947) definition of health that states, "health is a state of complete physical,

TABLE 2.2 A Comparison of Modern Practice Concepts and Nightingale's Canons for Health

Practice Concept	Canons
Physical environment	Ventilation and warming
	Light
	Cleanliness of rooms and walls
	Health of houses
Comfort and safety	Noise
	Bed and Bedding
	Personal cleanliness
Psychological Environment	Variety
	Chattering hopes and advices
Nutrition	Taking food
	What food?
Continuity of care	Petty management
	Observation of the sick

mental and social well-being, not merely the absence of disease or infirmity" (p. 29).

Nightingale's view of health separates the concepts of health and wellness. Wellness is an absolute state that may be more accurately described as being one end of the wellness-illness continuum. Although it might be difficult to define parameters that would place an individual on this continuum, it would be theoretically possible to do this. Therefore one would be more or less well, depending upon a variety of measurable factors.

Health, however, connotes a relative state. When defined as "being the best one can be at any given point in time," it allows an individual to be healthy even if not well. This statement relates to "using every power we have to use" (Nightingale, 1859/1949, p. 26).

By Nightingale's definition of health, an individual dying of cancer could still be in a healthy state, providing issues such as coping mechanisms, support systems, pain management, and grief support were provided. Yet this individual could hardly be considered well.

Nightingale's view of health included the idea that health was promoted by discovering the Natural Laws that govern health. By altering the environment according to Nightingale's canons, the

Natural Laws would be fulfilled and therefore, health would be promoted.

Nightingale (1893/1949) defined disease as "Nature's way of getting rid of the effects of conditions which have interfered with health" (p. 26). These conditions usually related to the effects of "dirt, drink [impure water], diet, damp, draughts [drafts], [and] drains [improper sewage disposal]" (p. 31).

Disease was also defined as a "reparative process" (1893/1946, p. 5). Viewing disease as "dys-ease," that is, lack of comfort, assists the reader in understanding Nightingale's viewpoint of health and illness. It is helpful to remember that during Nightingale's lifetime the vast majority of illnesses and deaths were caused by infectious disease. Therefore common symptoms would include fever, vomiting, nausea, diarrhea, and cough.

Each of these symptoms causes a level of discomfort or "dys-ease." However, they are therapeutic in the sense that each indicates a problem that exists within the body. Fever, for instance, only becomes nontherapeutic when not controlled. In most instances it does appear to be a natural way of ridding the body of the effects of illness. Therefore in this context, fever would be reparative.

Nursing

Nightingale viewed nursing as both an art and a science. The purpose of nursing was to "put the patient in the best possible condition for nature to act upon him" (Nightingale, 1859/1946, p. 6). Nursing was carried out by altering the environment in such a fashion as to implement the natural laws of health.

Nursing was viewed by Nightingale in both a general and specific context. In the general sense nursing was something carried out by women (as previously quoted from *Notes on Nursing*). Women who provided care in a family setting but had no formal training in nursing practiced "health nursing" or "general nursing."

Nightingale believed that women generally were poorly educated in how to care for their family's needs. When condemning the high mortality rate of infants she said:

Is all this premature suffering and death necessary? Or did Nature intend mothers to always be accompanied by doctors? Or is it better to learn the piano-forte than to learn the laws which subserve the preservation of offspring? (Nightingale, 1893/1949, p. 7)

In a specific sense, Nightingale envisioned "nursing proper" as that which was practiced only by women who had been educated as nurses (Nightingale, 1893/1949). This philosophical stance caused her to see the need for formalized nursing education and to work to establish the Nightingale School at St. Thomas' Hospital.

Nightingale's writings related to nursing care suggested that this care be carried out in a manner similar to what is now known as the "nursing process," even though Nightingale was not familiar with this terminology. Client observation was particularly important to the nursing process. It was a skill that she felt should be taught in an organized fashion to educated nurses.

Following observations, Nightingale felt that documentation of the observations should be made in detailed fashion. Organized record keeping resulted in the first nurses' notes. Emphasis was given to the environmental factors that the nurse was responsible for overseeing and altering, such as noise, light, and warmth.

Nightingale's Model of Nursing

Nightingale's model of nursing describes how a nurse is to implement natural laws. This model describes how these laws allow the concepts of person, environment, health, and nursing to interact.

All nursing must take place in the context of society and environment. While the nurse and the patient may be in the same environment, it is assumed that the alteration of the environment is for the improvement of the health of the patient. Certainly, it is clear that the context of 19th century England and the social values attached to the period had a profound effect on how Nightingale developed nursing.

Central to the nursing act is the person or patient who is the recipient of nursing care. Nightingale was very explicit that the person, not the disease, was to be nursed. The individual who is the recipient of nursing care may be ill or well, as the maintenance and promotion of health is as important as recovery from disease.

The model is linear. In this form the nurse is the active participant in the relationship. The outcome is the health state of the patient.

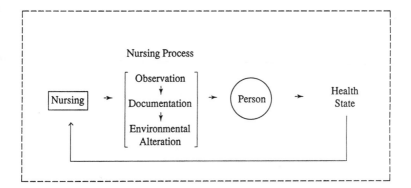

Figure 2.3. Nightingale's Model of Nursing Practice

This combination of process and outcome serves as feedback and indicates whether or not the nurse needs to modify nursing activities.

Nightingale did not see nursing as an event that only took place in the event of illness or injury; rather, Nightingale identified that nursing could take place as health promotion and rehabilitation activities, as well as in the restorative phase of illness.

Health promotion was a new concept at the time of Nightingale. She carried through with these beliefs by establishing district nursing—a precursor to public health nursing. Its purpose was to promote hygienic practices for the purpose of maintaining health.

Evaluation of Nightingale's Model of Nursing

Nightingale's model of nursing is based on experiential observations made about the relationship of individuals known as patients and their attendant health status. The health of individuals can be altered by manipulating the environment in such a fashion as to create more positive conditions for the patient. The individual who manipulates the environment is the nurse. The nurse would accomplish this manipulation of the environment through knowledge gained by observation and study.

In using observation as the major route to determining the relationship between the client and health, Nightingale employed inductive reasoning, a process by which one moves from a specific set of facts to determine a set of generalizations (Fitzpatrick & Whall, 1983). Nightingale was particularly adept at this method. Her experiences in the Crimea supplied her with the critical set of events and observations. From this experience she was able to identify patterns of change that needed to take place in the environment in order to increase patient well-being.

The model has been in actual practice settings for more than 100 years. Although nurses may not actually recognize that they are practicing nursing according to the Nightingale model, the goal of nursing action is frequently to alter the environment for the purpose of improving patient welfare. This flexibility indicates that it is a generalizable model.

The model is descriptive in nature (Fawcett, 1984). Although Nightingale described certain types of sequelae from patient environmental conditions, she never attempted to describe a causal relationship as to why these sequelae existed. For instance, she described that the lack of light produced rickets in children, and thus argued that light must be in the environment, but Nightingale never attempted to explain why a lack of light produced rickets.

Nightingale's theory is also simple. She does not attempt to define complex relationships between the elements of the theory. The simplicity does not seem to detract or reduce the theoretical applicability of the nursing practices that she describes.

Nightingale's theory may be classified as a grand theory (Fawcett, 1984). The theory has very broad terms and is abstract. This causes some difficulty in applying empirical testing to Nightingale's methods because the terms are imprecisely defined.

Perhaps the greatest testament to Nightingale's concepts of nursing is related to their durability. Although written well over a century ago, they are difficult to dispute and easy to apply even in today's high-tech health care settings.

3

Nightingale Then and Now

Is the study of Florence Nightingale and her perceptions of nursing merely an exercise in nursing history or does it have relevance for today's complex, high-tech world? The study of Nightingale proves to be basic to the present study of nursing practice.

Clinical Examples

Nightingale's emphasis was on providing an environment that would allow Nature either to heal or prevent illness. In virtually every modern nursing situation, regardless of the specific setting, the nurse remains responsible for altering the environment to improve it for the benefit of the client.

Case One

Mr. Wright, a gerontological nurse, has just completed a nursing assessment of Mr. Webster in his apartment. Mr. Webster is 90, lives alone, and has limited mobility. He depends on Social Security as his source of income. His son lives out of state. Although he is supportive of trying to meet his father's needs, he is rarely able to visit.

The apartment has adequate space but is poorly heated. The windows are painted shut and the apartment has a musty odor. The rooms have obviously not been cleaned for a long time. Moldy food is in the refrigerator.

As part of his nursing intervention, Mr. Wright arranges for a neighbor to clean the apartment on a regular basis. A fan is purchased to help with ventilation. Meals-On-Wheels provides at least one warm meal and daily contact with Mr. Webster. Mr. Wright contacted Mr. Webster's son and requested that on his next visit he see that Mr. Webster be provided with warmer clothing in order to try to maintain his body temperature during the upcoming winter.

Case Two

Mrs. Sanchez is caring for Nancy, a 16-year-old primipara who is in the first stage of labor. Having been admitted to the hospital 12 hours previously, Nancy appears tired and close to tears. Her contractions are every 2 to 3 minutes apart, lasting 45 seconds and are of moderate intensity. Nancy's mouth appears dry and her lips are cracked. She is sweating profusely. No family or friends are present.

In attempting to make Nancy more comfortable, Mrs. Sanchez encourages Nancy to walk in the hallway. She offers her ice chips, a lollypop, and lip lubricant. When she's in bed, Nancy's lower back is massaged. Mrs. Sanchez bathes Nancy's face and upper extremities and provides peri care. During contractions, Mrs. Sanchez helps Nancy focus her breathing to reduce her discomfort. As a result of these measures Nancy relaxes and is fully dilated within 45 minutes.

In each instance, the nurse manipulated the environment in some manner to benefit the client. In the case of the laboring mother, it is probable that the environment of both the mother and child was improved. The nursing actions are consistent with Nightingale's perception of nursing practice.

Nightingale Today

The real benefit of Florence Nightingale for today's practice is the legacy of values that she conferred upon modern nursing (Selanders,

1990). Much of what is taken for granted today—the clean environment for practice, the defined education, the movement of nursing toward an independent identity—is assumed to be the current standard. The origin of the standard rests with Florence Nightingale. Shealy (1985) has called Nightingale an example of an evolutionary personality because she redefined at least a portion of the universe as it was commonly understood to exist.

Nightingale's perceptions of nursing can be empirically tested as they relate to the modern nursing situation. Skeet (1980) has updated *Notes on Nursing: What It Is and Is Not* using Nightingale's original topic headings. Skeet demonstrated that these headings remain applicable in today's world of practice in *Notes on Nursing: The Science and the Art*.

Dennis and Prescott (1985) undertook a similar task by developing a qualitative database of current nursing practice, utilizing Nightingale's standards, in a contemporary setting. These standards were found to be applicable in modern practice.

Henry, Woods, and Nagelkerk (1990) demonstrated how Nightingale used principles of nursing administration to enhance nursing practice. Further examples exist in clinical studies in which Nightingale has been chosen as the organizing framework.

The strength of Nightingale's work lies partially in the durability of the ideas that she established over a century ago. Although she should be viewed neither as a saint nor seen as invincible, the utility of her principles of practice and education need to be remembered, used, and continually evaluated against the current standard.

Nightingale and Standards of Nursing Practice

Standards of nursing practice are criteria that were developed to allow for the evaluation of care against a known standard. The current criteria were developed by The American Nurses' Association (ANA) and are based on the nursing process (ANA, 1973). If Nightingale's theory is to serve as a model for current practice, then the theory should be able to withstand evaluation against these standards of practice.

Standard 1: Assessment

The collection of data about the health status of the client/patient is systematic and continuous. The data are accessible, communicated, and recorded.

Nightingale originated the concept of organized patient assessment. Further, she established assessment as a standard of nursing practice. In *Notes on Nursing*, she devoted extensive space to the process of observation. In it Nightingale (1859/1946) stated:

> The most important practical lesson that can be given to nurses is to teach them what to observe—how to observe—what symptoms indicate improvement—what the reverse—which are of importance—which are of none—which are the evidence of neglect—and what kind of neglect. All this is what ought to make part, and an essential part, of the training of every nurse. (p. 59)

Nightingale insisted that observations be made of individual patients to allow for individual variation. Routines and preferences of the patients were to be taken into consideration.

Recording of the data was also considered a critical component of nursing function. Record keeping grew out of Nightingale's Crimean experiences. Through thorough data collection and documentation she was able to support her perceived problems with the health care system. On a less global basis, the individual nurse was also expected to be able to write down observations and be able to support conclusions regarding prescribed care.

Standard 2: Nursing Diagnosis

Nursing diagnoses are derived from health status data.

Nightingale was not aware of the terminology of nursing diagnosis. Yet she freely drew conclusions regarding patient status from the data that she collected.

Today, nursing problems are frequently classified by nursing diagnoses. The North American Nursing Diagnosis Association (NANDA) has developed a list of nursing problems—actual, potential, or possible—with which the nurse may need to intervene.

A taxonomy of nursing diagnoses has produced a further ordering of nursing problems. NANDA has approved human response patterns as the accepted taxonomy. These categories include ex-

changing, communicating, relating, valuing, choosing, moving, per-
ceiving, knowing, and feeling (Kozier et al., 1991).

The problems listed in "Pattern 1: Exchanging" are primarily
physiological in nature. This pattern includes such functional categories as air exchange and elimination. Many of these areas were
directly or indirectly addressed by Nightingale, such as nursing care
for diarrhea, altered nutrition, hypo- and hyperthermia, ineffective
airway clearance, and potential for poisoning (Nightingale, 1859/
1946).

Standard 3: Planning

The plan of nursing care includes goals derived from the nursing
diagnosis.

Standard 4: Planning

The plan of nursing care includes priorities and the prescribed
nursing approaches or measures to achieve the goals derived from
the nursing diagnoses.

The prioritization of problems indicates that decisions must be
made as to how to approach and in what order to approach the
problems of a given patient. This ordering of decisions is reflected
in Nightingale's prioritization of problems with basic physiological
needs being the most important.

During Nightingale's lifetime the primary diseases that caused
sudden death were infectious. Common symptoms of fever, diarrhea, vomiting, and dehydration were frequently life threatening.
Consequently these problems required priority intervention. This
prioritization is also a reflection of the empirical process by which
Nightingale derived her nursing model.

Nightingale's definition of nursing—placing the patient in the
best condition for nature to act—implies that the very nature of
nursing is goal directed. In order to achieve the basic goal of nursing, more immediate goals must be designed by the nurse.

Standard 5: Implementation

Nursing actions provide for client/patient participation in health
promotion, maintenance, and restoration.

In Nightingale's paper presented at the 1893 Chicago Exposition, she stated:

> Health is not only to be well, but to be able to use well every power we have. . . . Both kinds of nursing [nursing proper and health nursing] are to put us in the best possible conditions for nature to restore or to preserve health—to prevent or to cure disease or injury. . . . Nursing proper is therefore to help the patient suffering from disease to live—just as health nursing is to keep or put the constitution of the healthy child or human being in such a state as to have no disease. (1893/1949, p. 26)

This definition of health is notable because it represents the first time that levels of health promotion, maintenance, and restoration were identified as being legitimate nursing functions. These functions of nursing remained essentially intact for a century until expanded and refined by reformers such as Virginia Henderson in 1955 (Furukawa & Howe, 1990).

Standard 6: Implementation

The nursing actions assist the client/patient to maximize health capabilities.

The goal of this standard is consistent with Nightingale's interpretation of health: that health is a relative process and involves helping the patient to be the best that he or she can be at any given point in time. Nightingale assumed that much of nursing care was done *to* the patient as opposed to in conjunction *with* the patient. Recipients of health care were not viewed as participants in the process. However, this view is assumed to be cultural and a function of 19th century ideology.

Standard 7: Evaluation

The client/patient's progress or lack of progress toward goal achievement is determined by the client/patient and the nurse.

As stated above, the patient frequently was not seen as an active participant in care. However, Nightingale did determine that the evaluation of client status was critical to the process of providing adequate care. Only then could it be determined if the care should be continued or altered.

Standard 8: Evaluation

The client/patient's progress or lack of progress toward goal achievement directs reassessment, reordering of priorities, new goal setting, and revision of the plan of nursing care.

This standard implies that the nursing process is circular in nature: As care is given, the assessment process begins again to redetermine the patient status. This process is consistent with the linear model representing Nightingale's practice of nursing. A feedback loop exists that provides the nurse with information about the outcome of care. Care is then altered accordingly.

It is an understatement to say that Nightingale's model of nursing practice is consistent with the *Standards of Nursing Practice* as established by the American Nurses' Association (1973). It is as if Nightingale's documents served as the basis for establishing these standards.

The Legacy of
Florence Nightingale

Florence Nightingale is recognized first and foremost as a nurse. She demonstrated skill as a social reformer and in creating change. What, then, is the legacy that has been left to the modern nurse?

Nightingale's skill in nursing was not at the bedside; rather, she was an administrator and reformer. Relative to the reform of nursing, she wrote:

> The whole reform of nursing both at home and abroad has consisted of this: to take the power over nursing out of the hands of the men and put it into the hands of one female trained head and make her responsible for everything being carried out. (Baly, 1981, p. 213)

In seeking to implement these reforms, Nightingale felt that nursing must establish an educational base. The result was the establishment of the Nightingale School and the development of the "Nightingale Model" of nursing education.

The major features of the model emphasized a combination of classroom and clinical experiences. Textbooks specifically designed for nurses were utilized. Nurses taught nurses although lectures by physicians did occur. Nightingale conveyed to the directors of the school her basic wishes in terms of curriculum and practical experience.

However, much of what Nightingale had originally designed was not actually carried out in practice. The most significant alteration of Nightingale's wishes was the apprenticeship system of nursing education that evolved and remained well into the 20th century.

In return for service given for little or no pay the student received a "free" education. The result was that the nursing schools became dependent on training hospitals for financial resources. Consequently the hospitals began to control training schedules, frequently limiting time and experience in the classroom in favor of the manpower hours that could be garnered at little or no expense to the institution.

In addition to issues of training, this situation continued to make nursing more subservient than Nightingale had envisioned. As a result, nursing continues to have problems with image.

A work completed by Etzioni in 1969 concluded that nursing, social work, and teaching were occupations that could never enjoy the same status as medicine and law—the professions. This was due to shorter training and a lack of autonomy. Both of these factors led to a less legitimized status as viewed by other professionals.

Although these arguments may be dated and inaccurate, they underscore the type of image problems with which nursing has had to deal. These arguments also demonstrate that nursing has not done well controlling its own destiny.

Is this the fault of Nightingale? Perhaps. Nightingale demonstrated throughout her lifetime that she was a powerful person and capable of creating change. She also demonstrated that she had the ability to assume leadership roles.

If Nightingale is to be faulted it is from the perspective that she did not appear to empower other nurses to assume the same type of leadership role that she so easily assumed. However, the leadership that she exhibited and the methods that she successfully employed are available for examination.

This point is where the study of Nightingale becomes valuable. Learning the lessons that she offered provides nursing with a wealth of possibility—and a lasting legacy.

References

Adams, E. C., & Foster, W. D. (1981). Heroine of modern progress. In R. G. Hebert (Ed.), *Florence Nightingale: Saint, reformer or rebel?* (pp. 102-107). Malabar, FL: Robert E. Krieger.

Allen, D. R. (1981). Florence Nightingale: Toward a psychohistorical interpretation. In R. G. Hebert (Ed.), *Florence Nightingale: Saint, reformer, or rebel?* (pp. 64-86). Malabar, FL: Robert E. Krieger.

American Nurses' Association. (1973). *Standards of nursing practice.* Kansas City, MO: Author.

Baly, M. E. (1981). Florence Nightingales's influence on nursing today. In R. G. Hebert (Ed.), *Florence Nightingale: Saint, reformer or rebel?* (pp. 210-219). Malabar, FL: Robert E. Krieger.

Baly, M. E. (1988). *Florence Nightingale and the nursing legacy.* New York: Croom Helm.

Calabria, M. D. (1990, Summer). Spiritual insights of Florence Nightingale. *The Quest* (pp. 66-74).

Cook, E. (1913). *The life of Florence Nightingale* (2 vols). London: Macmillan.

Cope, Z. (1958). *Florence Nightingale and the doctors.* London: Museum Press.

Dennis, K. E., & Prescott, P. P. (1985). Florence Nightingale: Yesterday, today and tomorrow. *Advances in Nursing Science, 1*(2), 66-81.

Dickens, C. (1986). *Martin Chuzzlewit.* Suffolk, UK: Richard Clay. (Originally published in 1843)

Etzioni, A. (1969). *The semi-professions and their organization.* New York: The Free Press.

Fawcett, J. (1984). *Analysis and evaluation of conceptual models of nursing.* Philadelphia, PA: F. A. Davis.

Fitzpatrick, J., & Whall, A. (1983). *Conceptual models of nursing: Analysis and application.* Bowie, MD: Robert J. Brady.

Furukawa, C., & Howe, J. K. (1990). Virginia Henderson. In J. B. George (Ed.), *Nursing theories: The base for professional nursing practice* (3rd ed., pp. 61-78). Englewood Cliffs, NJ: Appleton & Lange.

Goldie, S. M. (1987). *I have done my duty: Florence Nightingale in the Crimean War 1854-56*. Manchester, UK: Manchester University Press.

Henry, B., Woods, S., & Nagelkerk, J. (1990). Nightingale's perspective of nursing administration. *Nursing & Health Care, 11*(4), 201-206.

Kalisch, P., & Kalisch, B. (1986). *The advance of American nursing* (2nd ed.). Boston: Little, Brown.

Keen, N. (1982). *Florence Nightingale*. Berby, UK: J. H. Hall.

Kozier, B., Erb, G., & Olivieri, R. (1991). *Fundamentals of nursing: Concepts, process and practice* (4th ed.). Menlo Park, CA: Addison Wesley.

Nightingale, F. (1946). *Notes on nursing: What it is and is not*. London: Churchill Livingstone. (Originally published in 1859)

Nightingale, F. (1949). *Sick nursing and health nursing*. In I. Hampton (Ed.), *Nursing of the sick, 1893* (pp. 24-43). New York: McGraw-Hill. (Originally published 1893).

Palmer, I. S. (1977). Florence Nightingale: Reformer, reactionary, researcher. *Nursing Research, 26*(2), 84-89.

Pickering, G. (1974). *Creative malady: Illness in the lives and minds of Charles Darwin, Florence Nightingale, Mary Baker Eddy, Sigmund Freud, Marcel Proust, and Elizabeth Barrett Browning*. London: George Allen & Unwin.

Schultz, H. J. (1992). *British history* (4th ed.). New York: Harper-Perennial.

Seaman, L. C. B. (1956). *From Vienna to Versailles*. London: Coward-McCann.

Selanders, L. C. (1990). An American perspective of the Nightingale legacy. *Nursing Practice, 3*(3), 24-25.

Selanders, L. C. (1992). *An analysis of the utilization of power by Florence Nightingale 1856-1872*. (No. 9310445). Ann Arbor, MI: University Microfilms.

Shealy, M. C. (1985). Florence Nightingale 1820-1910: An evolutionary mind in the context of holism. *Journal of Holistic Nursing, 3*(1), 4-5.

Skeet, M. (1980). *Notes on nursing: The science and the art*. New York: Churchill Livingstone.

Torres, G. (1990). Florence Nightingale. In J. B. George (Ed.), *Nursing theories: The base for professional nursing practice* (3rd ed., pp. 31-42). Englewood Cliffs, NJ: Appleton & Lange.

Veith, S. (1990). The recluse: A retrospective health history of Florence Nightingale. In V. L. Bullough, B. Bullough, & M. P. Stanton (Eds.), *Florence Nightingale and her era: A collection of new scholarship* (pp. 75-79). New York: Garland.

Vicinus, M., & Nergaard, B. (1990). *Ever yours, Florence Nightingale*. Cambridge, MA: Harvard University Press.

Walker, L. O., & Avant, K. C. (1988). *Strategies for theory construction in nursing* (2nd ed.). Englewood Cliffs, NJ: Appleton & Lange.

Widerquist, J. G. (1992). The spirituality of Florence Nightingale. *Nursing Research, 41*(1), 49-55.

Williams, G. (1987). *The age of miracles: Medicine and surgery in the nineteenth century*. Chicago: Academy Chicago Publishers.

Woodham-Smith, C. (1953). *Florence Nightingale 1820-1910*. New York: Atheneum.

World Health Organization, Geneva Switzerland, 1947.

Bibliography

Adams, E. C., & Foster, W. D. (1981). Heroine of modern progress. In R. G. Hebert (Ed.), *Florence Nightingale: Saint, reformer or rebel?* (pp. 102-107). Malabar, FL: Robert E. Krieger.

Agnew, L. R. C. (1958). Florence Nightingale: Statistician. *American Journal of Nursing, 58*(5), 664-665.

Allen, D. R. (1981). Florence Nightingale: Toward a psychohistorical interpretation. In R. G. Hebert (Ed.), *Florence Nightingale: Saint, reformer, or rebel?* (pp. 64-86). Malabar, FL: Robert E. Krieger.

American Nurses' Association. (1973). *Standards of nursing practice.* Kansas City, MO: Author.

Baly, M. E. (1988). *Florence Nightingale and the nursing legacy.* New York: Croom Helm.

Baly, M. E. (1990). Florence Nightingale and the establishment of the first school at St. Thomas's—Myth v reality. In V. L. Bullough, B. Bullough, & M. P. Stanton (Eds.), *Florence Nightingale and her era: A collection of new scholarship* (pp. 3-22). New York: Garland.

Barritt, E. R. (1973). Florence Nightingale's values and modern nursing education. *Nursing Forum, XII*(1), 6-47.

Bishop, W. J., & Goldie, S. (1962). *A bio-bibliography of Florence Nightingale.* London: Dawsons of Pall Mall.

Bolster, E. (1964). *The Sisters of Mercy in the Crimean War.* Cork, Ireland: Mercier Press.

Brook, M. J. (1990). Some thoughts and reflections on the life of Florence Nightingale from a twentieth century perspective. In V. L. Bullough, B. Bullough, & M. P. Stanton (Eds.), *Florence Nightingale and her era: A collection of new scholarship* (pp. 153-167). New York: Garland.

Calabria, M. D. (1990, Summer). Spiritual insights of Florence Nightingale. *The Quest* (pp. 66-74).

Cohen, I. B. (1984). Florence Nightingale. *Scientific American, 3*, 128-137.

Cook, E. (1913). *The life of Florence Nightingale* (2 vols). London: Macmillan.

Cope, Z. (1958). *Florence Nightingale and the doctors*. London: Museum Press Limited.

Dennis, K. E., & Prescott, P. P. (1985). Florence Nightingale: Yesterday, today and tomorrow. *Advances in Nursing Science, 1*(2), 66-81.

Dickens, C. (1986). *Martin Chuzzlewit*. Suffolk, UK: Richard Clay. (Originally published in 1843)

Etzioni, A. (1969). *The semi-professions and their organization*. New York: Free Press.

Fawcett, J. (1984). *Analysis and evaluation of conceptual models of nursing*. Philadelphia, PA: F. A. Davis.

Fitzpatrick, J., & Whall, A. (1983). *Conceptual models of nursing: Analysis and application*. Bowie, MD: Robert J. Brady.

Fuld Health Trust. (1990). *The nurse theorists. Portraits of excellence: Florence Nightingale* (Part 1). (VHS Videocassette). Oakland, CA: Studio III.

Furukawa, C., & Howe, J. K. (1990). Virginia Henderson. In J. B. George (Ed.). *Nursing theories: The base for professional nursing practice* (3rd ed.) (pp. 61-78). Englewood Cliffs, NJ: Appleton & Lange.

Goldie, S. M. (1987). *I have done my duty: Florence Nightingale in the Crimean War 1854-56*. Manchester, UK: Manchester University Press.

Grier, B., & Grier, M. (1978). Contributions of the passionate statistician. *Research in Nursing and Health, 1*(3), 103-109.

Henry, B., Woods, S., & Nagelkerk, J. (1990). Nightingale's perspective of nursing administration. *Nursing & Health Care, 11*(4), 201-206.

Huxley, E. (1975). *Florence Nightingale*. London: Weidenfeld & Nicholson.

Isler, C. (1981). Florence Nightingale: Rebel with a cause. In R. G. Hebert (Ed.), *Florence Nightingale: Saint, reformer or rebel?* (pp. 176-190). Malabar, FL: Robert E. Krieger.

Kalisch, P., & Kalisch, B. (1983a). Heroine out of focus: Media images of Florence Nightingale—Part I: Popular biographies and stage productions. *Nursing & Health Care, (4)*, 181-187.

Kalisch, P., & Kalisch, B. (1983b). Heroine out of focus: Media images of Florence Nightingale—Part II: Film, radio, and television dramatizations. *Nursing & Health Care, (5)*, 270-278.

Kalisch, P., & Kalisch, B. (1986). *The advance of American nursing* (2nd ed.). Boston: Little, Brown.

Keen, N. (1982). *Florence Nightingale*. Berby, UK: J. H. Hall.

Keith, J. M. (1988). Florence Nightingale: Statistician and consultant epidemiologist. *International Nursing Review, 35*(5), 147-150.

Kozier, B., Erb, G., & Olivieri, R. (1991). *Fundamentals of nursing: Concepts, process and practice* (4th ed.). Menlo Park, CA: Addison Wesley.

Monteiro, L. A. (1974). *Letters of Florence Nightingale*. Boston, MA: Boston University.

Monteiro, L. A. (1985). Public health nursing then and now: Florence Nightingale on public health nursing. *American Journal of Public Health, 75*(2), 181-186.

Newton, M. (1949). *Florence Nightingale's philosophy of life and education*. Unpublished doctoral dissertation, Stanford University, California.

Nightingale, F. (1852). *Cassandra*. London: MacMillan.

Nightingale, F. (1946). *Notes on nursing: What it is and is not*. London: Churchill Livingstone. (Originally published in 1859)

Nightingale, F. (1949). Sick nursing and health nursing. In I. Hampton (Ed.), *Nursing of the sick, 1893* (pp. 24-43). New York: McGraw-Hill. (Originally published 1893)

Nightingale, F. (1954). Nursing the sick. In L. R. Seymer (Ed.), *Selected writings of Florence Nightingale* (pp. 319-352). New York: Macmillan. (Originally published 1882).

Palmer, I. S. (1977). Florence Nightingale: Reformer, reactionary, researcher. *Nursing Research, 26*(2), 84-89.

Palmer, I. S. (1981). Florence Nightingale and the international origins of modern nursing. *Image, 13*, 28-31.

Palmer, I. S. (1983a). Florence Nightingale and the first organized delivery of nursing services. *American Association of the Colleges of Nursing*, pp. 1-14.

Palmer, I. S. (1983b). Nightingale revisited. *Nursing Outlook, 31*(4), 229-233.

Palmer, I. S. (1983c, August 3). Florence Nightingale: The myth and the reality. *Nursing Times*, 40-42.

Pickering, G. (1974). *Creative malady: Illness in the lives and minds of Charles Darwin, Florence Nightingale, Mary Baker Eddy, Sigmund Freud, Marcel Proust, and Elizabeth Barrett Browning.* London: George Allen & Unwin.

Riehl-Sisca, J. (1989). *Conceptual models for nursing practice* (3rd ed.). Englewood Cliffs, NJ: Appleton & Lange.

Schultz, H. J. (1992). *British history* (4th ed.). New York: Harper-Perennial.

Seaman, L. C. B. (1956). *From Vienna to Versailles.* London: Coward-McCann.

Selanders, L. C. (1990). An American perspective of the Nightingale legacy. *Nursing Practice, 3*(3), 24-25.

Selanders, L. C. (in press). *An analysis of the utilization of power by Florence Nightingale 1856-1872.* Ann Arbor, MI: University Microfilms.

Shealy, M. C. (1985). Florence Nightingale 1820-1910: An evolutionary mind in the context of holism. *Journal of Holistic Nursing, 3*(1), 4-5.

Showalter, E. (1981). Florence Nightingale's feminist complaint: Women, religion, and suggestions for thought. *Journal of Women in Culture and Society, 6*(3), 395-412.

Skeet, M. (1980). *Notes on nursing: The science and the art.* New York: Churchill Livingstone.

Strachey, L. (1988). *Eminent Victorians.* New York: Weidenfeld & Nicholson.

Torres, G. (1990). Florence Nightingale. In J. B. George (Ed.), *Nursing theories: The base for professional nursing practice* (pp. 31-42). Englewood Cliffs, NJ: Appleton & Lange.

Veith, S. (1990). The recluse: A retrospective health history of Florence Nightingale. In V. L. Bullough, B. Bullough, & M. P. Stanton (Eds.), *Florence Nightingale and her era: A collection of new scholarship* (pp. 75-79). New York: Garland.

Vicinus, M., & Nergaard, B. (1990). *Ever yours, Florence Nightingale.* Cambridge, MA: Harvard University Press.

Walker, L. O., & Avant, K. C. (1988). *Strategies for theory construction in nursing* (2nd ed.). Englewood Cliffs, NJ: Appleton & Lange.

Widerquist, J. G. (1992). The spirituality of Florence Nightingale. *Nursing Research, 41*(1), 49-55.

Williams, G. (1987). *The age of miracles: Medicine and surgery in the nineteenth century.* Chicago: Academy Chicago Publishers.

Woodham-Smith, C. (1953). *Florence Nightingale 1820-1910.* New York: Atheneum.

About the Author

Louise C. Selanders, Ed.D., R.N., is Assistant Professor of Nursing at Michigan State University in East Lansing, Michigan. She completed her doctorate in Educational Leadership at Western Michigan University in Kalamazoo, Michigan. Her research interests include nursing history, sociological issues of nursing education, and nursing administration.